Rock Steady
Cheers

FIGHTING PARKINSON'S WITH VOICE AND SPIRIT

PAUL D. BILLINGSLEY, DMin

ISBN (e-book) 979-8-218-09028-9

ISBN (softcover) 979-8-218-08998-6

Printed in the United States of America

With Special Thanks To My Coaches

Carol Edmiston

Who taught me how to become a fighter
against Parkinson's

Betsy Lerner

Whose energy in training taught me
the importance of endurance

Nic Kemps

Who gave me the first opportunity
to lead a group cheer

Kim Novosad

Whose resourcefulness and affirmation
encouraged me to write cheers

ABOUT THE AUTHOR

Paul D. Billingsley lives in Greensboro, North Carolina with his dog Higgins. Since being diagnosed with Parkinson's in 2019, he has made a strong commitment to exercise to keep Parkinson's at bay.

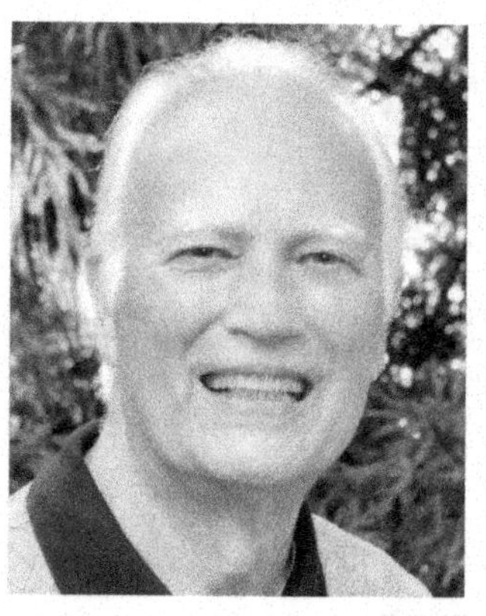

He is a member of Rock Steady Boxing at PurEnergy Fitness Center Greensboro where he is better known as Pirate Paul.

Cycling classes at Ragsdale Family YMCA are also an important part of his fitness strategy. Regarding posture, he trains with Prince Deece of A.C.T. by Deese.

For over 40 years he served churches in Texas and the Carolinas. He is a graduate of Southwestern Baptist Theological Seminary with Master of Divinity degree and New Orleans Baptist Theological Seminary with Doctor of Ministry degree.

INTRODUCTION

The cheer is a vital part of a Rock Steady Boxing® class. A cheer is a set of somewhat rhythmic words or phrases which relate to the class and the fight against Parkinson's.

Best suited for the end of a class, the concluding cheer is meant to send fighters away with a sense of togetherness and inspiration. While a cheer is often engaged by a group, it is also affirming when read aloud or spoken by an individual outside of class.

A good cheer will convey a simple truth or message. A humorous thought or phrase may be included from time to time. My initial experience of a class cheer was at the conclusion of my very first boxing class. The coach called participants into a close circle. Everyone was led to extend an arm toward the center of the circle. We then stacked hand upon hand.

Line by line the cheer was announced by the coach. After each line, everyone in the circle would echo what was just stated by the coach. The second rendition was much louder as everyone in the class participated. The class and concluding cheer were my first steps toward learning what it meant to be a Fighter.

For the last few moments of the class, I became one with the group. As with a shout, we lifted our hands off the stack and upward toward the ceiling, a sense of challenge and hope flushed my spirit. Not until later would I be ready to announce my name and say "I am a fighter". But the journey had begun.

The journey would not be made alone. Already new acquaintances were being enjoyed. We would chat at the water fountain during brief training breaks. A laugh might be shared to brighten energy demanding moments. We would encourage one another as we worked to give our best to completing exercises correctly. Every challenge urged by a coach was visibly met with tenacity.

These classmates were fast becoming friends. All of us came together because of a common adversary. We all were fighting back against Parkinson's. While each of us encountered unique PD experiences, we often shared similar life challenges. Our common aggressor pushed us to fight back. We were unique in experience yet we were much the same. We were all fighters.

egardless of the number of fighters in a class, we were one in spirit. This became more evident to me as we joined in a circle and a cheer. The cheer was the spoken spirit of Rock Steady Boxing®.

Then one class the coach announced, "After this exercise, Pirate Paul is going to lead us in a cheer." I think we all were a little surprised, although I was the most. Finishing the exercise, we moved into a circle and everyone extended an arm and hand toward the circle center.

Then, everyone turned and looked expectantly at me.

"Rock Steady is our friend

Rock Steady helps us bend

Rock Steady helps us win

Rock Steady Boxing!"

The cheer I lead and everyone repeated was simple, yet it worked. Class ended on a positive note.

We all had participated in a surprise conclusion. Because one of us had a winning experience, we all had won.

A cheer may express a fighter's own experience. Although brief, a facet of one's own story may be expressed in these few words. Though simple, the phrases of a cheer let light burst through bringing a sense of affirmation, victory, or renewed hope.

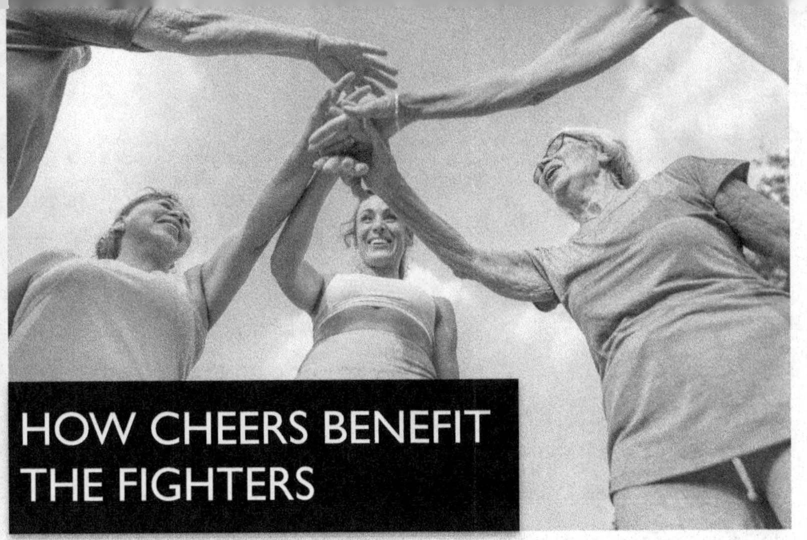

HOW CHEERS BENEFIT THE FIGHTERS

One way cheers benefit the fighter, is to give emphasis to verbal expression. This is significant because with a progression of Parkinson's, one may experience a loss of vocal strength. The voice becomes small. One loses the bigness or amplitude of their voice. Sometimes a person can hardly be heard even when only a few feet away.

When this occurs in a class, coaches will encourage fighters to increase voice volume or repeat what was just said, only louder. Exercises are included during classes which include big range of motion and away from smaller movement. Such have the added benefit of helping one maintain or build voice strength.

A cheer at the conclusion of a class allows fighters to join together with strong voice to end the class on a high note. When all join in an energetic cheer in the closing moments of a class, even the most tired fighter can leave the class inspired and with an inward smile. The cheer matters. By taking part, one can experience a spirit of finishing well. Indeed, the cheer is the spoken spirit of Rock Steady Boxing®.

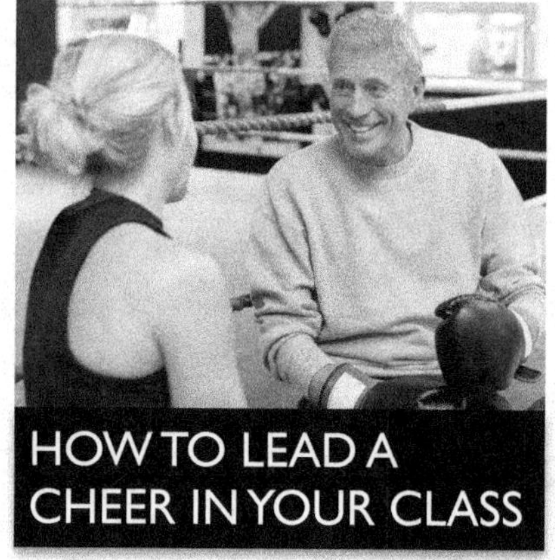

Typically cheers come at the end of a class. But cheers could be used at the beginning or during a class. Fighters usually are called to circle up close together and extend an arm and hand towards the center of the group circle. The Leader will do well to call out the cheer with a strong voice. This will call attention to the cheer, signify its importance, and guide the fighters to finish strong.

Remember the following:

1. Words should be announced clearly so all can make the correct response.

2. A brief explanation of the subject of the cheer may be helpful to alert fighters and get everyone ready to participate. Most often no such attention is needed.

3. Every cheer will be more effective if called with a sense of rhythm. Although each line of a couplet is rather short, be aware of the rhythm that best helps deliver the cheer.

4. Most cheers conclude with a two or three word refrain. For example, Rock Steady is an affirmation of challenge accepted, progress made, work accomplished, strength of purpose, a victory gained, or maybe settled determination.

The refrain Rock Steady Boxing® is the name of the organization and fitness program regardless of location. Repeating this refrain calls attention to the world-wide organization, affirms one's connection with purpose and mission of the organization, and brings unity in thought to conclude the class.

5. The refrain of the cheer should be called out with gusto. One arm should be lifted into the air with clinched hand while emphasizing the chosen refrain. Most will follow your lead, maybe all.

A cheer enables everyone to finish strong. The cheer lets every fighter participate in the spoken spirit of Rock Steady Boxing®.

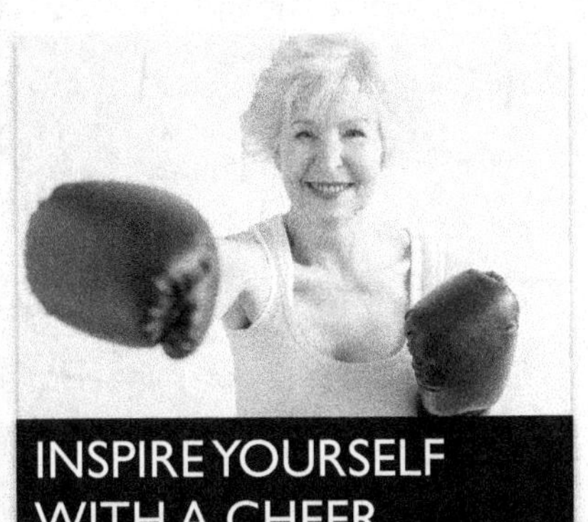

A cheer may be read or spoken aloud when one is alone. One does not have to be a class member to benefit from the spirit of the cheers. Although the cheers were born out of the experience in boxing classes, the genesis behind each cheer is the confrontation against Parkinson's.

One's own experience opens the heart to connect with a cheer. So, a cheer can bring personal encouragement and meaningful inspiration even when experienced outside of class. This can bring one hope for the journey. As a wise King said many years ago "A cheerful heart is good medicine." Proverbs 17:22 NIV

TABLE OF CONTENTS

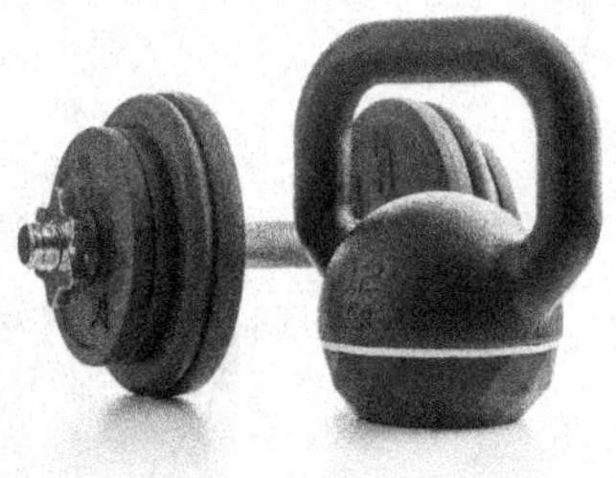

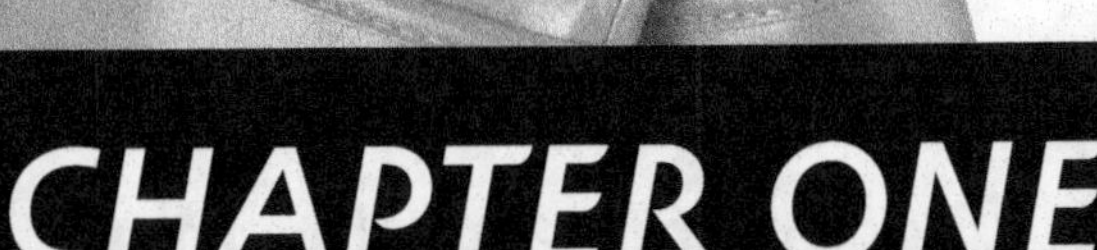

WE'VE GOT CLASS

One Class

One class at a time

Discipline becoming mine

Getting stronger every day

Training the Rock Steady way

Rock Steady Boxing!

Every day we have been given

Rock Steady helps us with the liv'n

To the classes I'll be sticking

Today I'm giving PD a licking

Rock Steady Boxing!

On My Mind

Got Rock Steady Boxing on my mind

Came to see what I would find

Learned to box and how to fight

How to punch PD with all my might

Rock Steady Boxing!

One Class Is Not Enough

Just one class is not enough

To beat PD or make one tough

Every class builds on the other

Finish one class be ready for another

Rock Steady!

First Day

First day I started on a mat

Warmed up for boxing on that flat

Then rolled up the mat, stood up tall

There was more to do, I did it all

Rock Steady!

Glad I Didn't Stay At Home

Glad I didn't stay at home

Although, at first, I felt like foam

Now I'm moving this way, that way

Rock Steady Boxing made my day

Rock Steady Boxing!

A New Start

Every class gives a new start

Fighters engage with strength and heart

We never know until the end

How far we've come how good its been

Rock Steady!

Boxing Class Is Just One Way

Boxing class is just one way

I'm staying active every day

Keeping my personal goal in sight

Fighting PD with all my might

Rock Steady Boxing!

Good Medicine

Rock Steady is good medicine

Helps us get through thick or thin

Does not matter how hard its been

Against PD we aim to win

Rock Steady!

Gives Me Punch

Boxing classes give me punch

Glad I'm part of this brave bunch

Throwing punches and guarding my face

I may become a fighting ace

Rock Steady Boxing!

The Right Schedule

Trying to get my schedule right

Some appointments hide from sight

Marked in red are all the days

Boxing class meets and gets my praise

Rock Steady!

A Fresh Start

Every class gives a fresh start

Challenges the mind and strengthens
the heart

When the clock signals class to end

We have new confidence to return again

Rock Steady!

Very Good Outlook

Came to class wondering if I could

If others can, surely I would

Now I'm boxing, as told I should

Thinking my outlook is very good

Rock Steady!

A Bold Fight

First class, thought I'd never make it

Second class, I improved a bit

Then I set a boxing goal

Now I'm fighting very bold

Rock Steady Boxing!

Before The Mirror

When we box before the mirror

Helps us see a little clearer

How much progress we have made

And that our training has really paid

Rock Steady!

Fighter Friends

What we're doing is very clear

Beating PD is why we're here

Working with our fighter friends

Our best is what the class commends

Rock Steady Boxing!

Exercise Wisdom

Our schedules sometimes keep us apart

Rock Steady Boxing stays in our heart

When we remember to exercise

We all know we are wise

Rock Steady Boxing!

Path To Victory

No two classes are the same

Variety makes us glad we came

So many ways to target PD

Each way a path to victory

Rock Steady Boxing!

Know What Helps

Know what helps all this shaking?

Be active, keep moving is the plan I'm taking

Joined Rock Steady, learned what to do

Helps my shaking, and thinking too

Rock Steady!

A Challenge Given

Parkinson's is a challenge I have been given

Rock Steady Boxing keeps me driven

To the classes I'll be sticking

Training to give PD a licking

Rock Steady Boxing!

Train With Friends

Training with my fighter friends

Against PD we must defend

Working out to build our cardio

Keeping us strong and on the go

Rock Steady Boxing!

Put On Gloves

Put on the wraps, put on the gloves

Greet everyone with a gentle glove shove

We know boxing is for our good

Going "all in" is just understood

Rock Steady Boxing!

Push Back

Every class offers moments of hope

Helping fighters do more than just cope

We are learning how to attack

Resisting PD we daily push back

Rock Steady Boxing!

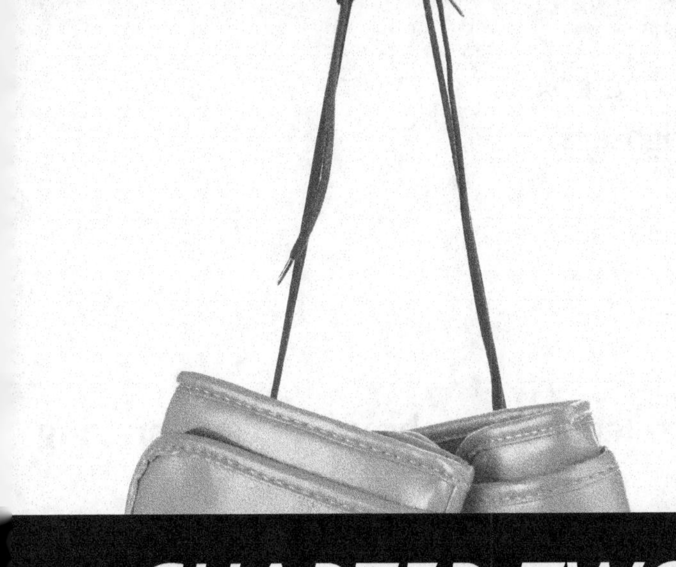

LEARNING TO BOX

True Fighters

We're learning to box but have no ring

No ropes, no lights, no bell to ding

Yet true fighters we each are

Training to pound PD when we spar

Rock Steady!

A Fight For Me

Learning to box is a fight for me

Each one's fight is unique you see

There is no fighting one another

The PD fight is something other

Rock Steady Boxing!

Our Fighting Ace

Boxing with a jab, cross, hook

Not always easy as it looks

Training to fight the foe we face

Boxing is our fighting ace

Rock Steady!

Training Is Hard

Training is hard, not much grinning

Especially when just beginning

Get a little stronger after a while

And returns the winning smile

Rock Steady!

Clever Like A Fox

Now I'm learning how to box

Getting clever like a fox

Although not ready for the ring

I give PD a loaded ding

Rock Steady Boxing!

A Challenging Fight

We're in a challenging fight

We learn to give it all our might

Yet it's necessary to relax

So our bodies we will not tax

Rock Steady Boxing!

Friends Who Understand

At first it was a rather odd feeling

Knowing it's PD with which I'm dealing

Joined boxing friends who understand

Learned to fight PD with my hands

Rock Steady Boxing!

The Heavy Bag

Learning to box surprised me

Did not know a fighter I could be

Now the heavy bag is my friend

In better shape than I have been

Rock Steady!

Met Some Boxers

Met some boxers, learned how to fight

Learned to box with all my might

Beating PD is why I train

Determined to have a victory campaign

Rock Steady Boxing!

Lots Of Stretching

Lots of stretching keeps me limber

Breathing helps, I must remember

Touch the ceiling, touch the wall

I get more flexible with every call

Rock Steady!

Taking Care To Stretch

Taking care to stretch the back

Better here than in the sack

Hold it, hold it, count to ten

More limber now than I have been

Rock Steady Boxing!

Flexibility Is Our Friend

Sometimes class starts on the floor

Stretching some, then stretching more

Warming up, so we can bend

We know flexibility is our friend

Rock Steady!

"Get To Know Ya"

In "Get To Know Ya" circles we learn much

What fighters do, like, and such

Then on our feet or on the floor

Stretch a lot, we know there's more

Rock Steady Boxing!

My Balance

Learning to box with no routine

Variety helps keep alive the dream

Building stamina to hold me steady

Balance and posture keep me ready

Rock Steady!

Stay Steady

Balance helps me to stay steady

Always alert, always ready

Hold it, hold it, count from ten

Hold without falling, then do it again

Rock Steady!

Tired To Inspired

When I feel a little tired

And my "want to" needs inspired

A little water, a moments rest

Helps me re-engage and give my best

Rock Steady!

Remembering Purpose

If I think I'm getting tired

Remembering purpose does inspire

Challenging me to do my best

Fighting PD to give it a rest

Rock Steady!

Needing A Cup Of Joe

If we enter class feeling low

Thinking we need a cup of Joe

After we become engaged with all

Leave feeling refreshed and walking tall

Rock Steady Boxing!

Determination Inside

Some days I don't feel like much

But I'm not looking for a crutch

It's what's inside that really counts

I've got determination in ready amounts

Rock Steady!

"Can Do" Power

Exercise gives us "Can Do" power

Helps us stand another hour

We may feel tired, but we won't quit

We know exercise makes us fit

Rock Steady!

Determination Inside

If my energy is running low

And determination needs to show

I think later will be time to rest

So now I'll give it all my best

Rock Steady!

Get Up And Go

Sometimes I feel like my "Get Up and Go"

Has got up and gone, but I know it's not so

Staying active really helps a lot

And I'm thankful for the "Go" I've got

Rock Steady!

What We Eat

Now I'm learning what's good to eat

Fruits and veggies are hard to beat

Sweets are tasty, but not really best

Nuts and beans are more likely blessed

Rock Steady Boxing!

Healthy Cuisine

If we watch what we eat

Veggies can make our diet complete

If we add meat, fruits, and beans

We can have healthy cuisines

Rock Steady!

Another Step

Today my training took another step

So glad I'm keeping up my pep

Boxing helps me stay strong and ready

Trains my balance keeps me steady

Rock Steady Boxing!

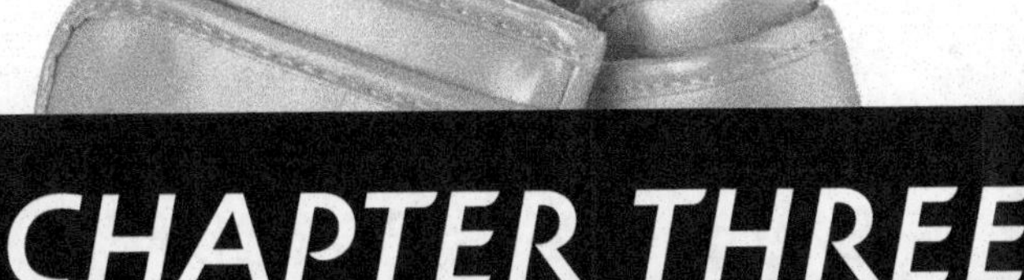

EXERCISE PILL

A Very Strong Pill

Today may be the very day

Exercise holds PD at bay

Staying active honing my skills

Finding exercise a very strong pill

Rock Steady!

Proper Execution

There is no substitution

For proper execution

Each exercise makes a contribution

To building up one's constitution

Rock Steady!

Aerobic Exercise

Aerobic exercise makes me sweat

Grab a towel no need to fret

Do it again, ten times, then twenty

Do it right, there's hope aplenty

Rock Steady!

Developing Muscles

Developing muscles, one aim of training

Strength and agility is what we're gaining

We're all different, yet much the same

Pushing back PD is why we came

Rock Steady Boxing!

Hear Our Voices

Hear our voices when on the mat

Arch the back, scream the cat

Extend the stomach, bellow the cow

Use big voice when strength allows

Rock Steady!

Work At Home

When the gym closes the door

Work at home can help us more

When we remember to exercise

We all learn that we are wise

Rock Steady!

No Couch Potato

No more acting like a couch potato

No more feeling like a rotten tomato

Gotta keep active every day

Keep moving and smiling all the way

Rock Steady!

A Self Ovation

After the dust has settled

And class has tested my mettle

I gain a winning sensation

I'm giving me a self ovation

Rock Steady!

Mixing Exercises

When we mix our exercises

Works very well for all our sizes

There's no wonder and no doubt

Beating PD is what it's all about

Rock Steady!

Put On Gloves

Put on gloves and box a while

Seems much better than running a mile

Starting in the boxing stance

Jab, cross, hook, and I'll advance

Rock Steady!

Working Hard

Working hard and staying steady

Moving strong and always ready

Staying active and physically fit

Targets PD for a robust hit

Rock Steady!

Repetition

Exercise is better when done correctly

I will get it right directly

Repetition is building strength in me

Keeping me fit to punch PD

Rock Steady!

Sing Your Song

Exercise keeps the body young

Puts songs in the heart to be sung

Everyone sings in their own key

The tunes I sing strengthen me

Rock Steady!

Fighting Stance

Got my outfit, gloves, and wraps

In boxing you don't need a cap

Fighting stance gets special attention

Punching PD is my intention

Rock Steady!

EXERCISE PILL
Staying Active

Staying active is a key

In our fight against PD

So we exercise every day

And our health we won't betray

Rock Steady!

The Music Beat

Music helps fighters move our feet

We do exercise to the beat

Hearing music from earlier days

Our memory and timing can amaze

Rock Steady!

Flatten Abs

Today we stretched to get ready

To flatten our abs, tighten our belly

It takes more than the planks we do

We also climb a mountain or two

Rock Steady!

Learning To Exercise

Learning how to exercise

Staying active is very wise

Training hard to defeat PD

Making a fighter out of me

Rock Steady Boxing!

EXERCISE PILL
Rest Later

When I feel I'm getting tired

And I need to be inspired

I think later will be time to rest

So now I'll give it all my best

Rock Steady Boxing!

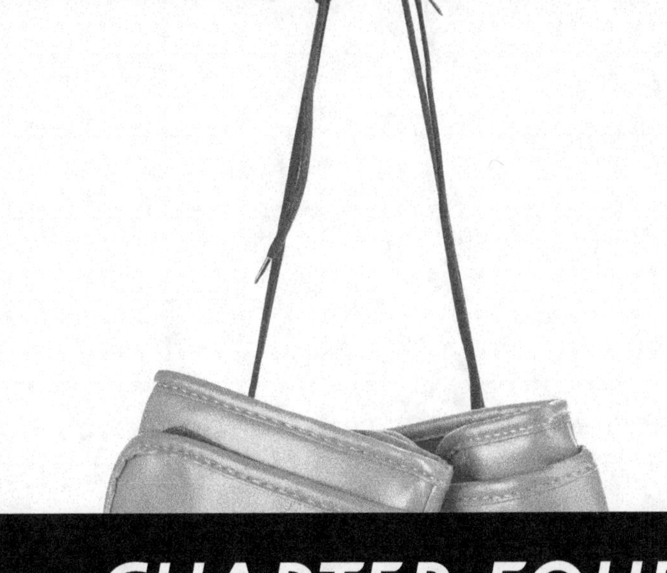

CHAPTER FOUR

WE ARE FIGHTERS

Fight Like Bears

When we fighters put on the gloves

Someone may think we look like doves

Not one of us really cares

When we fight, we fight like bears

Rock Steady!

A Fighter Is Born

Once my tennis shoes were new

Been to a lot of classes, not a few

Even my shoe laces now are worn

Look at me, a fighter is born

Rock Steady!

A Battle To Fight

We each have a battle to fight

Our challenge is heavy, not light

The PD enemy must give way

To the fighter, able and ready today

Rock Steady!

We are fighters, we attack

Nothing gained by holding back

Hit the bag harder, do your best

Those big gloves not made to rest

Rock Steady!

Mighty Fighters

We are fighters, we all train

Friends together, none complain

We work hard to get it right

Close to us you'll sense our might

Rock Steady!

Wake Up Call

Giving my strength a wake up call

Gonna give this fight my very all

A Rock Steady spirit pushes me

Determination engages me totally

Rock Steady!

Courageous Fighters

We are fighters, our courage is strong

We fight Parkinson's all day long

We remember if we feel alone

There's a boxing family to which we belong

Rock Steady Boxing!

We are fighters, we train hard

Our name is on the PD card

In this battle, we push back

Determined and ready to attack

Rock Steady!

Dancing Fighters

We are fighters, looking to advance

Can't believe we had to dance

Left foot, right foot, so it goes

Turn and finish with a fighting pose

Rock Steady!

One For All

We are fighters, we all are

Friends together, not one star

One for all, and all for one

When one wins, we all have won

Rock Steady!

I'm A Fighter

I'm a fighter, we learn to say

Against PD there's no other way

And it's becoming truer every day

Against PD "I'm a fighter" all the way

Rock Steady!

We Train As One

Coming together, we train as one

My way, your way, we get it done

Developing skills, how we've grown

We are fighters, that's how we're known

Rock Steady!

No Shortcuts

It takes brains and it takes guts

We work hard and no short cuts

We look tough and we're the best

We fight PD to give it a rest

Rock Steady!

A Daily Fight

Never thought I'd have this feeling

I now know it's PD with which I'm dealing

So it's a fight I'm daily giving

I'm determined to give PD a licking

Rock Steady!

Honor The Name

We are fighters that's our claim

We work hard to honor the name

We give our best and there's no shame

Striving for better, never stay the same

Rock Steady!

One Unique Band

One by one the fighters came

Each one different, yet much the same

Finding friends who understand

One heart, one hope, one unique band

Rock Steady Boxing!

Stand Tall

Exercise helps me to stand tall

Keeps me walking and on the ball

Helps my balance I'm glad to know

Builds me up, keeps me on the go

Rock Steady Boxing!

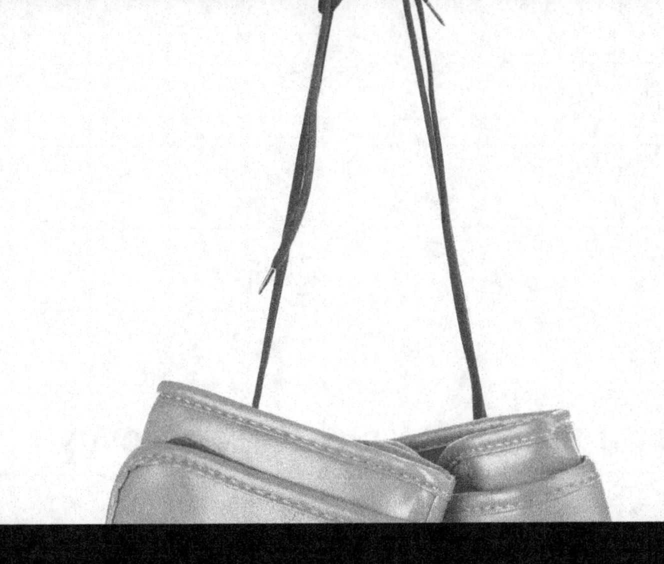

CHAPTER FIVE

FINISH STRONG

Big Finish

Put on the wraps, put on the gloves

Greet all with a gentle glove shove

Knowing what we do is for our good

Working for a big finish is just understood

Rock Steady!

Final Minute

When the clock points to the final minute

Persistence has brought me to be in it

Giving PD another blemish

End the class with a big finish

Rock Steady!

Leave Your Mark

Fighting PD is no walk in the park

Some days it is swimming with the sharks

Exercise and boxing gives one heart

To punch PD and leave your mark

Rock Steady!

Getting In Shape

Getting in shape is hard to do

Staying in shape is very hard too

So we remember one prize and goal

Being healthy and strong when we're old

Rock Steady!

Finish Strong

Every class holds something new

There are challenges, not a few

We train together all class long

When we're through we finish strong

Rock Steady!

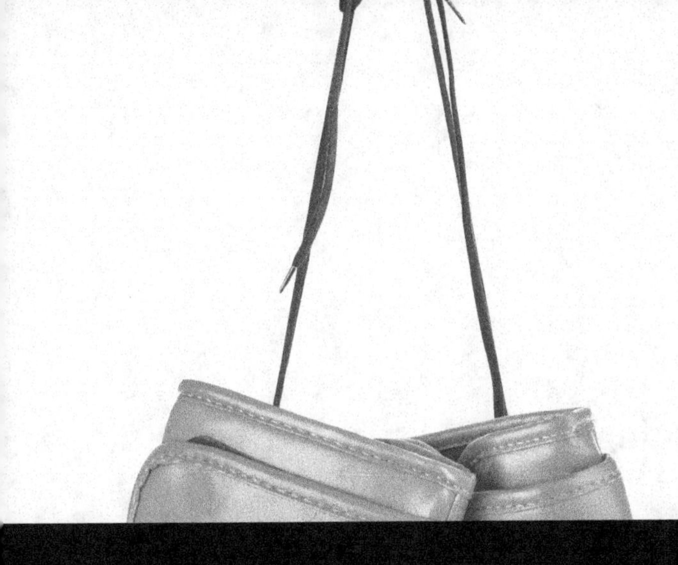

WE'VE GOT HOPE

Fighting PD

Fighting PD was little known to me

Now it's a daily fight I see

Rock Steady gives a helping hand

Offers me hope for the fights demand

Rock Steady!

Moments Of Hope

Defeating PD is the goal at hand

Vigorous exercise is part of the plan

There's always a prayer to help us cope

Looking up we find moments of hope

Rock Steady!

Together In The Fight

We're all together in this fight

Working out together gives us light

Training together we increase our might

Friendship together keeps hope in sight

Rock Steady!

I Belong

To Rock Steady, I belong

The exercise we do makes us strong

Repetitive training is real dope

Maintaining fitness gives us hope

Rock Steady!

Extended Power

Exercise gives me extended power

Builds endurance for the hour

If ever temptation comes to quit

Hope rises and renews my grit

Rock Steady!

Faces Speak

The faces I see speak to me

We're all in a struggle with PD

There's a lot of challenge in the fight

Every win keeps hope in sight

Rock Steady!

Energy Level

One's energy level can be revealing

When its PD with which we're dealing

Exercise raises one's hope of progressing

And determination to see PD regressing

Rock Steady!

Hard Thinking

Today I'm doing some very hard thinking

From this PD fight I'm not shrinking

Friends encourage along the way

With an earnest prayer it's a hope filled day

Rock Steady!

Determination

A cheer may tell a PD story

Challenge & commitment, not much glory

The words remind us how we've been

How determination brings us hope again

Rock Steady!

Hope Abounds

Today class took a lot of energy

It won't be lunch until a nap for me

Taking a deep breath I look around

We all are fighters and hope abounds

Rock Steady!

Hope Wins

Today I gave it all I've got

Think I may drop on this spot

Can't believe all I've done

Go home tired, but hope has won

Rock Steady!

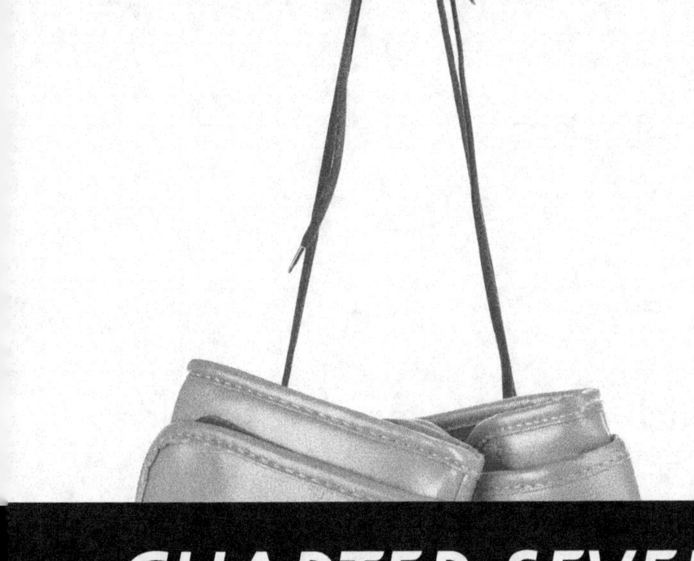CHAPTER SEVEN

COACHES
SAY

Coach Is Looking

Coach is looking over my shoulder

I'm training harder, a little bolder

Strength flames from an energy smolder

Now I'm my own record holder

Rock Steady!

Do Your Best

When we gather with boxing friends

We challenge each other to better ends

Coaches help us to achieve

We do our best when we believe

Rock Steady!

Getting Better

Class is finished another day

"Getting better" coaches say

But I'm feeling a little sore

Glad I'm headed out the door

Rock Steady!

"Break for water" coaches say

Stay refreshed along the way

"Don't forget to breathe" they tell

So we can reach the final bell

Rock Steady!

Build Muscles

Working out can be inspiring

Building muscles is what we're desiring

Coaches challenge us to do our best

It's up to us to do the rest

Rock Steady!

Exercise Is Good

Coaches say "Exercise is good"

Early on I understood

Words can be very cheap

But in doing, strength takes a leap

Rock Steady!

COACHES SAY
Channel Your Strength

I'm getting stronger every day

"Channel your strength" the coaches say

When focused energy gets it right

Repetition builds up my might

Rock Steady!

Guided By Coach

I'm a fighter we always say

We mean it more every day

Guided by our coaches plans

We learn there is power in our hands

Rock Steady!

Hit It Harder

The heavy bag does not complain

Hit it harder, there's so much to gain

Hold your posture, get it right

Building strength for the PD fight

Rock Steady!

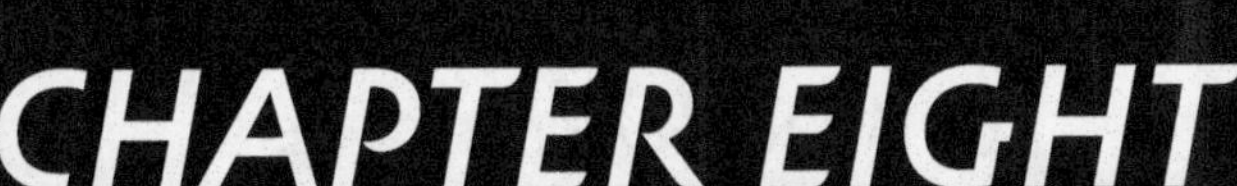

ON THREE

Beat PD on three

One, Two, Three

Beat PD!

Punch PD on three

One, Two, Three

Punch PD!

Pound PD

Pound PD on three

One, Two, Three

Pound PD!

Rock Steady Boxing on three

One, Two, Three

Rock Steady Boxing!

Finish Strong

Finish Strong on three

One, Two, Three

Finish Strong!

Knock out PD on three

One, Two, Three

Knock Out PD!

Strong Fighter

Strong fighter on three

One, Two, Three

Strong Fighter!

Rock Steady on three

One, Two, Three

Rock Steady!